KATHERINE WHITE

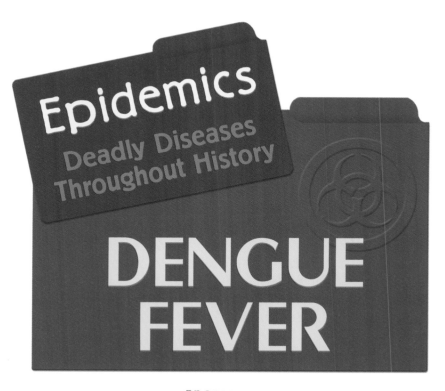

Epidemics
Deadly Diseases
Throughout History

DENGUE FEVER

The Rosen Publishing Group, Inc.
New York

The author would like to thank Mark Bender for sharing the story of his personal experience with dengue fever.

Published in 2004 by The Rosen Publishing Group, Inc.
29 East 21st Street, New York, NY 10010

Library of Congress Cataloging-in-Publication Data

White, Katherine, 1975–
Dengue fever / by Katherine White.
    v. cm. — (Epidemics)
Includes bibliographical references and index.
Contents: What is dengue fever?—Early history and epidemics—Researching treatments, handling outbreaks—Prevention and the future.
ISBN 0-8239-4200-7 (libr. bdg.)
1. Dengue—Juvenile literature. [1. Dengue. 2. Diseases. 3. Epidemics.] I. Title. II. Series.
RC137 .W476 2003
616.9′21—dc21

                                        2003000730

Manufactured in the United States of America

Cover image: A colorized image of dengue fever particles

CONTENTS

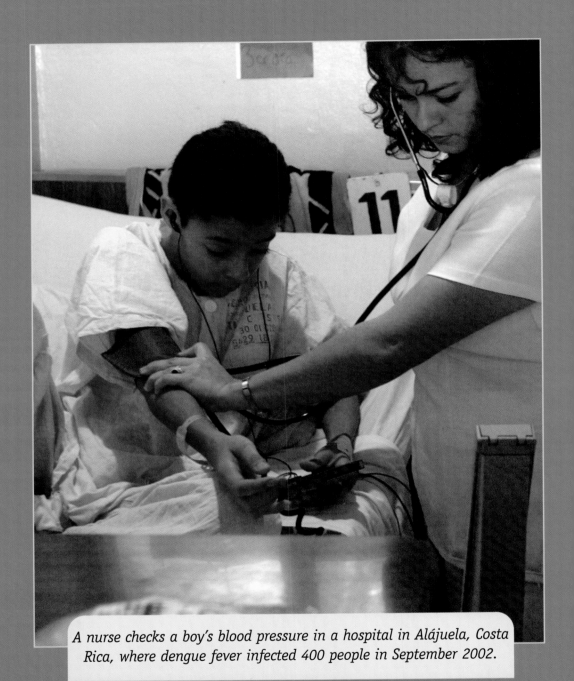

A nurse checks a boy's blood pressure in a hospital in Alájuela, Costa Rica, where dengue fever infected 400 people in September 2002.

INTRODUCTION

Dengue fever, also known as breakbone fever, is making headlines all over the world. On August 29, 2002, the *Wall Street Journal* ran the article, "Dengue, Asian Fever, Is Spreading," which reported a large number of dengue fever infections during recent years. The huge leap in dengue cases is causing many scientists and medical experts to worry.

Dengue fever is a mosquito-borne illness, which means it is spread to a person through a mosquito's bite. The disease also thrives in tropical environments, so warm, damp climates are being overrun with dengue. Dengue fever is quickly spreading through Southeast Asia in places like Bangkok, Kuala Lumpur, Malaysia, and Singapore. It has also been seen in Hawaii and

Texas. According to the *Wall Street Journal*, "In late July, the World Health Organization (WHO) issued a warning about dengue, estimating that there are 50 million cases a year and that 2.5 billion people in 100 countries, or 40 percent of the world's population, are potentially at risk."

This is not the first time dengue fever has made the news. In AD 265 to 465, a Chinese encyclopedia of diseases, symptoms, and remedies included a disease called water poison. Then, people thought this "water poison" disease was connected with flying insects and water. Now, scientists view this entry as what might be the first medical acknowledgment of dengue fever. The symptoms of water poison were similar to dengue—high fever and bone and joint pain.

If dengue has been around for so many years, why are scientists worrying now? Medical experts believe the disease may start a new phase because infections are rising so fast. Statistics are showing new and larger epidemics than ever before. In Rio de Janeiro alone, dengue may have affected around 500,000 people. The WHO also estimated 400,000 cases of dengue hemorrhagic fever in Southeast Asia in 2001. In the United States, Hawaii had a new outbreak from May 2001 to February 2002, the first in many years.

Dengue fever is at epidemic proportions and the numbers are still climbing. An epidemic is a disease that affects a large number of individuals within a population, community, or region at the same time.

Right now, there is no cure for dengue fever. In fact, one of the biggest challenges the medical community faces is how to control and contain dengue— how to stop the disease from spreading. Even though dengue is not fatal, many scientists and experts are searching for a cure. A cure is the best way to contain this threatening disease.

1

WHAT IS DENGUE FEVER?

The Centers for Disease Control and Prevention (CDC) is an organization that monitors and gathers facts and information on all the diseases affecting the world's population. The CDC's job is to learn as much as possible about a disease. The CDC's main goal is to lower a person's risk of contracting, or getting, any disease. If many people become ill, the CDC also works to contain the virus or disease, so other people do not become infected. Right now, the CDC is monitoring dengue fever quite closely. The organization posts important updates on its Web site to inform medical experts as well as the public about dengue fever and the new places where the disease has cropped up.

Four Different Viruses

As reported by the CDC, dengue fever is caused by four closely related but distinct viruses. An example of the virus would be the one that causes the common cold you have probably had more than a few times.

Dengue fever is actually caused by four different viruses that are incredibly similar; they are called virus serotypes. A virus serotype is a scientific term for a closely related virus that shares similarities. In other words, virus serotypes are very much alike. Dengue fever virus serotypes are:

- DEN-1
- DEN-2
- DEN-3
- DEN-4

Not all of dengue's serotypes were discovered at the same time. DEN-1 and DEN-2 were discovered in 1960. The DEN-3 strain of dengue was discovered in 1961, while DEN-4 was discovered in 1963.

DEN-1, DEN-2, DEN-3, and DEN-4 are so closely related that the only way to find out which strain a person has is to get a blood test. Even then scientists find it hard to identify which of the four virus serotypes a person is carrying. This means each serotype mirrors the other serotypes so closely that symptoms and progression follow almost the same pattern.

In science and medicine, every disease belongs to a system that compares one disease to another. This system organizes diseases so that doctors, scientists, and medical experts can understand how every disease is similar to and different from one another. This system of classification is known as taxonomy.

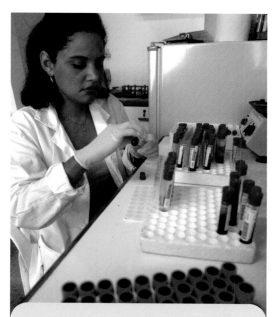

A doctor checks blood samples for traces of dengue fever during an outbreak in Costa Rica in 2002.

The four serotypes of dengue fever belong to the genus *Flavivirus*, family Flaviviridae. There are three major illnesses caused by Flaviviridae: tick-borne encephalitis virus, Japanese encephalitis, and dengue fever.

Getting Dengue More Than Once

A person can get dengue fever four times in his or her lifetime, although a person never gets the same dengue infection twice. Infection with one type of dengue fever provides immunity for the rest of a person's life. Immunity is when a person cannot become infected with a virus he or she has already carried. How then can a person get dengue more than once?

Each dengue strain is unique, so that a person can be potentially infected once by each strain of the virus. Forunately, it is very rare that a single person is unlucky enough to contract four dengue infections.

Transmission

Dengue fever is transmitted to humans by the bite of an infected mosquito. Transmission means the virus is being passed or spread to someone else.

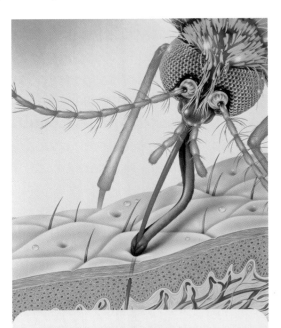

An illustration of a mosquito piercing the skin of its human victim.

When a mosquito bites a person, some of its own blood mixes with the human it is biting. If that mosquito is infected with dengue fever, the mosquito's blood will be transmitted into the human's blood via a small hole made by the mosquito's needle-like tongue. When the infected blood mixes with the human's blood, a person is infected with dengue fever. Mosquitoes initially get dengue fever when they bite a dengue-infected person. The mosquito is then capable of spreading the disease to anyone it bites. There is evidence that shows the *Aedes aegypti* mosquito is able to pass dengue fever to its offspring as well.

The *Aedes aegypti* is dengue's transmitter, or the mosquito that most commonly spreads dengue fever, in the Western Hemisphere. Countries like the United States, Canada, Venezuela, Barbados, Mexico, Cuba, and Guatemala are part of the Western Hemisphere.

The *Aedes aegypti* Mosquito

Adult *Aedes aegypti* mosquitoes like to rest indoors and feed, or bite people, during the day. There are two peaks in their feeding: early morning for two to three hours and then in the afternoon for a few hours before dark. The female mosquito feeds differently from the male because the female tends to be more nervous while feeding. Any small movement from a person interrupts the female mosquito's feeding. However, she will return only a few moments later, time and time again.

The female *Aedes aegypti* often infects a few people in the same household because she does not have her

The Harvard School of Public Health reports some interesting facts about mosquitoes.

- Mosquitoes are found worldwide across all temperature zones.

- They comprise more than 2,500 species.

- Mosquitoes are weak fliers but may fly as far as 1 to 1.5 miles in one hour.

- Malaria (another mosquito-borne illness) kills more than 1 million people annually.

- Thousands of hairs on the mosquito's antennae can sense moisture, lactic acid, carbon dioxide, body heat, and movement.

- A female mosquito takes a nap after having a blood meal to assist in the digestion process.

entire meal in one long bite. Instead, she has a few small bites to complete her meal.

The book *Dengue and Dengue Hemorrhagic Fever*, edited by D. J. Gubler and G. Kuno, describes *Aedes aegypti* as a small, black-and-white mosquito. *Aedes aegypti* prefers to lay its eggs in places like the containers found in and around people's homes. Flower vases, buckets filled with old rainwater, unused tires, and soggy trash are all breeding grounds for this mosquito. Water storage containers like big cement drums or septic tanks are big enough for mosquitoes

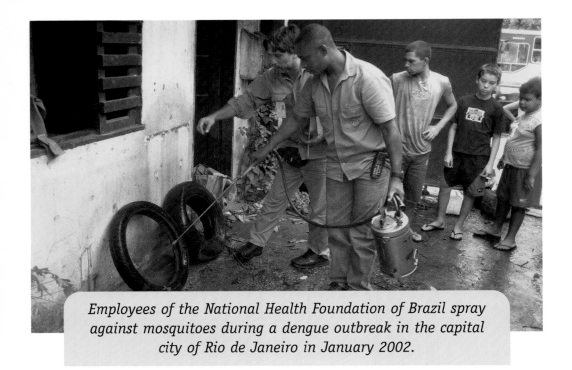

Employees of the National Health Foundation of Brazil spray against mosquitoes during a dengue outbreak in the capital city of Rio de Janeiro in January 2002.

to breed in larger numbers. Unfortunately, most of these places are usually close to cities, homes, and people, so many mosquitoes have a high chance of coming into contact with people and infecting them.

So what makes the tropics the hot zone for dengue fever? It actually has everything to do with the characteristics of a tropical climate. Areas of continuously hot and humid weather mixed with an abundance of rain make perfect breeding grounds for mosquitoes. In the tropics, mosquitoes can also breed all year round. This increases the number of mosquitoes, and it also increases the ability of one infected mosquito to breed hundreds more.

Mosquito Life Cycle

According to the American Mosquito Control Association, there are more than 2,500 species of mosquitoes throughout the world. But most mosquitoes develop in the same way. There are four stages in the mosquito's life cycle: egg, larva, pupa, and adult.

Egg

The *Aedes aegypti* lay their eggs on damp soil that will be flooded by water. Eggs are laid one at a time or attached together to form rafts, which float on the surface water. Most eggs hatch into larvae within forty-eight hours.

Larva

Water is a necessary part of the mosquito's life, so the larva lives in the water and comes to the surface to breathe. Larvae look like small centipedes. Some mosquitoes breed in specific habitats, such as ponds or salt marshes. As long as the water is stagnant though, like in barrels, the larvae can and will survive.

Pupa

The pupal stage is a resting, nonfeeding stage of development. It is also the stage in which the mosquito changes into an adult. Much like a butterfly comes from a cocoon, the pupal skin splits and an

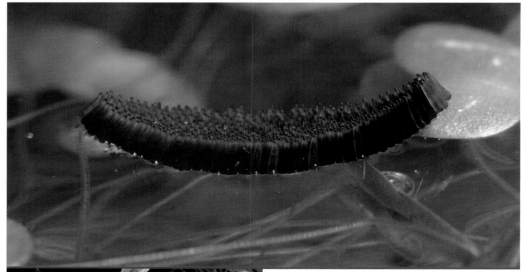

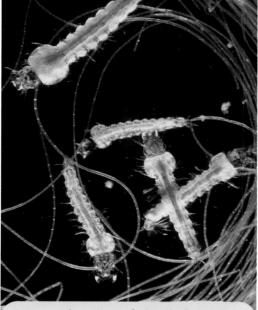

A mosquito egg raft (top) floats in a pool in Oxfordshire, England. Mosquito larvae (bottom) are shown at the water's surface.

adult mosquito emerges. This stage takes between two to four days.

Adult

The adult mosquito stays on the surface of the water for a brief time to dry and let all of its body parts harden. Blood feeding and mating do not happen for a couple of days. A mosquito's life span can vary from one week for males to several months for females.

Symptoms of Dengue Fever

Dengue fever is known for having a variety of symptoms, all of which happen after a sudden high fever. The fever ranges from 102°F to 105°F (38.8°C to 40.5°C), and it may last for two to seven days. Other symptoms of dengue are:

- severe headache
- backache
- joint pain
- nausea and vomiting
- mild sore throat
- eye pain
- full body rash, including face, hands, and feet
- general weakness

Hemorrhaging, or bleeding, is also not uncommon with dengue fever. Bleeding can be mild or severe. Bleeding of the gums and gastrointestinal (stomach and intestines) bleeding are the most common forms of hemorrhaging.

Most of the time, dengue fever is transmitted to older children and adults, meaning very young children are rarely infected with dengue. If a younger child does become infected, he or she almost always has a milder illness than older children and adults.

Viral Progression and Treatment

Dengue and Dengue Hemorrhagic Fever reports, "After a person is bitten by an infective mosquito, the virus undergoes an incubation period of three to fourteen days (average, four to seven days)." An incubation period is the time from the moment of exposure to the development of the symptoms of the disease.

Currently, dengue fever has no treatment and no cure. Medical experts and scientists are studying possible cures, but there is little evidence that one will be discovered soon. Dengue is not fatal, meaning it is very rare that anyone dies from the disease. However, a person with dengue fever should always see a doctor. If he or she is feeling extremely ill, seeking immediate medical attention at a hospital is definitely advised.

Medical professionals treat dengue patients with rest, and they make sure the patient gets plenty of fluids. Beyond those basics though, the patient has to let the virus runs its course.

Dengue Hemorrhagic Fever

Dengue hemorrhagic fever, or DHF, is a more severe form of dengue fever. This type has the same symptoms as dengue fever, but it advances into a more severe case faster. In fact, DHF can be fatal if it goes unrecognized or is improperly treated. DHF mostly affects children under the age of fifteen. The WHO estimates that 20 million cases occur each year, requiring 500,000 hospitalizations.

DHF is a complication of dengue fever. It is different from dengue in that the patient may lose so much blood due to hemorrhaging that he or she can go into shock. This is why it is considered a more serious sickness than dengue fever and why DHF gets its own name. There is some evidence that being infected with different dengue serotypes increases the risk of DHF.

DHF is caused by the same viruses that cause dengue fever. Early on, it also has the same symptoms as dengue. Tests cannot even distinguish the difference in the first few days of the disease.

There are three stages of DHF:

Stage 1

Like dengue fever, dengue hemorrhagic fever begins with a fever that lasts from two to seven days. The infected person also experiences the same signs and symptoms that could occur with many other illnesses, including dengue fever.

Stage 2

The next stage of DHF is the forming of hemorrhagic manifestations, which simply means the patient begins to bleed. Bruises are made easily, and as with dengue fever, the patient may bleed from the nose or gums. In rare cases, the patient begins to bleed internally, and the smallest blood vessels begin to leak.

Stage 3

The circulatory system fails, followed by shock. In most cases, death follows if the circulatory failure is not stopped. DHF is fatal in only 5 percent of patients.

Understanding Dengue Fever

Dengue fever and DHF are on the rise. In order to further understand dengue fever, scientists are studying the pattern of its development. They have already answered some major questions about the virus, such as how it spreads and where it thrives. The hope is that the more scientists learn about dengue, the closer medical scientists can move toward a cure. The next chapter chronicles the history of dengue fever—its epidemics and pandemics and how the disease spreads. You'll be interested to know humans helped spread the disease to many new parts of the world.

2

HISTORY AND EPIDEMICS

Dengue fever has a long history. The disease has created hundreds of epidemics and pandemics, affecting millions of people throughout the world. A pandemic occurs when a disease spreads over a wide geographic area and affects an exceptionally large number of people. Epidemics and pandemics are similar because they both involve a disease or sickness that affects a region or population. A pandemic is different than an epidemic, though, because the area of sickness is larger and more spread out, which usually means more people fall sick.

Interestingly, people and their various modes of transportation played one of the most significant roles in dengue fever's spread. When boat travel became popular, travelers on large ocean liners actually brought dengue fever from the Tropics to the United States. The disease was eventually spread to non-tropical cities such as Philadelphia, Pennsylvania, and Austin, Texas.

Dengue's Early Years

The Pan American Health Organization (PAHO) timeline of dengue fever marks 1635 as the year dengue most likely created its first stir. In this case, dengue was identified in Martinique and Guadeloupe, two islands in the Caribbean. It then fell silent, resting quietly until 1779 or 1780, when the disease began to explode. Scientists then saw dengue in North America, Asia, and Africa. In 1780, a dengue-like disease caused an epidemic in Philadelphia.

Philadelphia is not a tropical environment, but dengue was being spread to different regions of the world. The shipping of goods, called imports and exports, was becoming more popular, and the *Aedes aegypti* mosquito was going along for the ride. Ships were actually carrying the mosquito to new lands, and once there, the mosquito would begin to breed. Consequently, dengue fever would crop up.

Epidemics and Pandemics

The first medically confirmed dengue epidemic came in 1818 when Peru was struck with 50,000 dengue cases. Soon after came a pandemic in and around the Caribbean from 1827 to 1828. A pandemic occurs when a disease spreads over a wide geographic area and affects an exceptionally high number of people.

In this case, dengue first affected the Virgin Islands. It then crawled slowly west to Cuba, Jamaica, and Venezuela. At the same time, mosquitoes and infected travelers were being carried to various locations around the world by ships. People fell sick in Pensacola, Florida; Charleston, South Carolina; Savannah, Georgia; and New Orleans, Louisiana. Most of these infected places are port cities—they are found along a coastline. This makes for humid, damp, and moist climates—perfect weather for mosquito breeding. Next, dengue moved into Veracruz, Mexico, where it disappeared in 1828.

Pandemic and Epidemics: 1845–1900

In 1845, dengue cases were reported in St. Louis, Missouri, and Rio de Janeiro, Brazil. By 1846, Brazil had an epidemic on its hands, and by 1850, so did many southern United States cities. New Orleans, Savannah, and Charleston were under siege with dengue fever. The virus also broke out in Brownsville, Texas; Augusta, Georgia; Woodville, Mississippi; and Mobile, Alabama.

The end of the nineteenth century found dengue fever all over the world. From 1870 to 1900, dengue cases were reported anywhere from New Orleans to the Caribbean. In fact, 40,000 people were infected with dengue in New Orleans in 1870. There was also an epidemic in the Caribbean and the southern United States from 1879 to 1880 as well as the first outbreak in the Bahamas in 1882.

Only three years later in 1885, Austin and other nearby Texas towns faced an epidemic. This time, between 16,000 and 22,000 people fell sick. However, this was only a prelude to the terrifying epidemic in 1897 when almost every city and village across the state of Texas was affected by dengue. The southern United States and the Caribbean were again faced with an epidemic from 1897 to 1899.

Twentieth-Century Pandemics

The turn of the century did not slow dengue epidemics. Instead, the disease remained on a steady incline. According to the PAHO timeline, dengue outbreaks and flare-ups played a major role in the first twenty years of the twentieth century.

- 1904 Cases reported in Florida, Texas, and Panama

- 1905 Cases reported throughout the Caribbean

- 1907 Cases from the Mississippi to Colombia and Cuba

⊗ 1912 Cases reported in Panama

⊗ 1914 Cases reported in Iquique, Chile

⊗ 1915 Epidemic in Puerto Rico

⊗ 1916 Cases reported in northern Argentina

⊗ 1916 Epidemic in Brazil

The 1920s brought more dengue cases and an explosion of dengue outbreaks. In 1921, there was an outbreak in the Bahamas that lasted for one year. Then in 1922 came one of the largest epidemics of dengue in the history of the United States. In Texas, between 500,000 and 600,000 people were infected. There were 30,000 people infected in Galveston, Texas, alone.

From 1922 through 1924, Louisiana also struggled with dengue fever, although on a much smaller scale. In 1922, 7,561 people were affected, and in 1923, 1,376 people fell ill. Fortunately, by 1924 the spread of dengue halted with only one person becoming infected the entire year.

In 1923, Rio de Janeiro, Brazil, was also battling an epidemic that took about a year to control. But just as dengue began to spread, it simply disappeared. For twenty years, dengue was silent, leaving scientists baffled as to why the disease stopped. To this day, scientists are not sure why the disease dropped off quietly and no longer cropped up. They think that a

AD 265 to 465	1635	1780
A Chinese encyclopedia of diseases, symptoms, and remedies includes a dengue-like disease called water poison.	A disease similar to dengue fever appears in Martinique and Guadeloupe in the Caribbean.	A disease that mirrors dengue fever causes an epidemic in Philadelphia, Pennsylvania.

change in weather patterns may have had something to do with the sudden decrease, but no study has ever figured out the exact reasons.

World War II and Dengue: 1939 through the 1950s

When World War II broke out in 1939, soldiers from all over the world were shipped to Europe through 1942. War shipments of weapons and food, even uniforms, were also moved from place to place. Again, dengue fever was spread around the world by humans, especially in Southeast Asia and around the Pacific Ocean.

1827–1929
The First known pandemic breaks out in the Virgin Islands, Jamaica, Cuba, and Venezuela (Caribbean-Gulf-Atlantic region).

1851–1853
An epidemic plagues Brazil.

1879–1880
The Caribbean and the southern United States suffer an epidemic.

1897
An epidemic occurs in Texas, the Caribbean, and the southern United States.

(continued on page 28)

From 1941 through 1946, there were epidemics in the Caribbean, Mexico, Panama, Venezuela, and Texas Gulf cities. There were cases reported in Puerto Rico, Bermuda, Cuba, and the Bahamas. World War II also provoked a huge wave of DHF, the more dangerous form of dengue fever.

The first epidemic of DHF happened in Manila, Philippines, from 1953 to 1954. In the next twenty years, the disease would spread throughout all of Southeast Asia in epidemic proportions. By the middle of the 1970s, DHF was one of the biggest causes of hospitalization and death of children in and around Southeast Asia.

1921–1922
An outbreak takes place in the Bahamas

1941–1946
An epidemic spread through the Caribbean, Mexico, Panama, Venezuela, and Texas Gulf cities

1968–1969
Dengue epidemic in the Caribbean and Venezuela.

1975
Puerto Rico suffers a dengue epidemic.

The 1960s and Beyond

In 1958, the Pan American Sanitary Conference Resolution was held. The goal of the meeting was to encourage countries to work toward the eradication of dengue fever. Eradication meant getting rid of dengue fever completely. The conference asked ten countries and territories to increase their anti-dengue activities. Belize, Bolivia, Brazil, Ecuador, French Guiana, Nicaragua, Panama, Paraguay, Peru, and Uruguay all agreed to fight dengue fever.

Due to eradication efforts, there were not many dengue epidemics during the 1960s and the early

1990
DEN-1 appears in in Ecuador

2000
A DEN-1 outbreak plagues Paraguay.

2001–2002
Hawaii endures a dengue epidemic.

1996
DEN-3 is reported in Costa Rica, Guatemala, Honduras, and Mexico

2002
Dengue fever hits Rio de Janeiro.

1970s. In fact, in twenty-one countries the *Aedes aegypti* mosquito had been mostly eradicated, especially in Central and South America. But, when eradication programs ended in the early 1970s, dengue and DHF again reinfected the same countries. Without prevention, there was no hope for control.

From 1971 to 1972, around 500,000 people fell sick with dengue fever in Colombia. This area had not seen dengue fever since 1952. Then, in 1972 to 1973, Puerto Rico battled a small epidemic, around 7,000 cases.

The end of the 1970s found most of the high-risk countries battling dengue in one form or the other. Between 1977 and 1980, dengue fever was cropping up in huge numbers. In 1977, an epidemic began in Jamaica that would affect 400,000 people in three years. The epidemic then spread to Cuba, where it created a huge wave of viruses in one year: 477,440 cases were reported in 1977. From Cuba, dengue fever spread into the Bahamas and then into Antigua, Aruba, Barbados, Barbuda, Curaçao, Dominica, the Dominican Republic, Grenada, Guadeloupe, Guyana, Haiti, Martinique, Montserrat, Puerto Rico, St. Kitts, St. Martin, St. Vincent and the Grenadines, Trinidad, Turks and Caicos, and the Virgin Islands. The total estimate of dengue cases was around five million people.

By the 1980s, Central and South America were again experiencing epidemics in some places that had not seen dengue for 35 to 130 years. For example, in March 1986, Rio de Janeiro experienced its first dengue outbreak since 1923. By the time the epidemic ended a few months later, more than two million people had become ill with the virus, and a new threat had come to light. Brazil, for the first time, had a death toll from dengue fever. Now, Brazil was not only up against dengue fever but also dengue hemorrhagic fever as well.

A similar thing happened in Venezuela from 1989 to 1990. Although this was Venezuela's second outbreak of DHF, DEN-1 and DEN-2 were now also present. Unfortunately, the next decade brought more

Prepared by the World Health Organization, the table below shows the world's dengue fever (and DHF) statistics from 1998 to 2001. As can be seen, 1998 was a big year for dengue fever.

CASES	1998	1999	2000	2001
Western Pacific	356,554	64,066	45,603	N/A
Southeast Asia	218,859	55,405	57,997	119,707
Americas (DF)	708,146	317,040	394,847	400,875
Americas (DHF)	12,426	5,216	5,667	5,331
Americas (total)	720,572	322,256	400,514	406,206
Eastern Mediterranean	0	0	0	0
Africa	0	0	0	0
World	1,295,985	441,727	504,114	525,913

of the same trend. During the 1990s, countries that had been infected with only one virus serotype in the past became infected with two or three of them. The scientific term for a country that is infected with more than one dengue serotype is hyperendemicity.

Current and Recent Outbreaks

In the past, dengue fever came in waves, with outbreaks occurring in large groups. In the past ten or fifteen years, dengue fever has once again exploded in the same way. But why? Many leading scientists cite two main causes: A huge growth in population and uncontrolled growth of cities. Many times newer cities are not designed well, so they have poor water, sewer, and waste management systems. All of these make for incredible mosquito breeding.

Dengue Hits Hawaii

From May 2001 to February 2002, Hawaii was on alert. For more than a few months, dengue had been cropping up in Maui. Alerts were made to travelers to be careful when visiting Maui in hopes of decreasing infection. During February, health officials became worried because heavy rains could have drastically increased mosquito breeding. What worried health officials the most, however, is that Hawaii had not seen dengue fever since World War II. At that time, 1,500 people became ill and the city of Waikiki was actually closed! In this recent case, the epidemic was not nearly so large. Only 119 people fell sick with dengue.

Rio de Janeiro Epidemic

Around January 2002, dengue fever began to explode in Rio de Janeiro. According to a February 26, 2002, article in the *New York Times*, "The number of cases exceeded 100,000 just in the state of Rio de Janeiro, and smaller outbreaks were reported elsewhere." The disease had struck pop stars, soccer players, and almost the entire cast of a popular soap opera. The

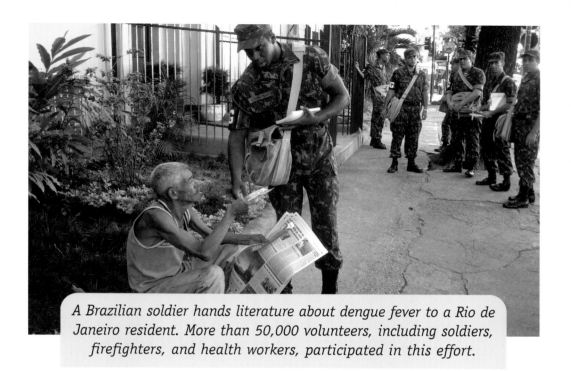

A Brazilian soldier hands literature about dengue fever to a Rio de Janeiro resident. More than 50,000 volunteers, including soldiers, firefighters, and health workers, participated in this effort.

sudden epidemic had quite an impact. Health officials recommended that people stay away from Tijuca, one neighborhood where infections were exceptionally high. In Brazil, there have been 317,787 cases of dengue fever including 57 deaths, with Rio de Janeiro being the most affected area; 41 percent of all the dengue cases came from there. Overall, Rio de Janeiro's dengue cases were up 886 percent from 2001.

By April 25, 2002, the Pan American Health Organization reported, "95,463 cases in Rio de Janeiro, including 571 dengue hemorrhagic fever (DHF) cases and 31 deaths." Luckily, this was a big decrease, representing only 3 percent of cases reported since the beginning of the epidemic.

3

RESEARCHING TREATMENTS, HANDLING OUTBREAKS

One of the most challenging aspects of dengue fever is that scientists are not close to finding a cure. Another tricky aspect of the disease is that so few people actually know about it. Travelers go to new places not even knowing dengue fever exists, making them completely vulnerable to the sickness.

Mark Bender, a network analyst in Chicago, knows firsthand about dengue fever. Over the Christmas holidays in 1998, while still a sophomore at Penn State University, Bender became infected with dengue fever while vacationing in Australia. Before getting dengue fever, Bender had never even heard of it. In a recent interview, he said he will never forget it.

Q. Where were you traveling when you got dengue fever?

A. I was traveling in Port Douglas, Australia. It is a small town on the northeast coast of Australia located within the tropical rain forest region of Queensland.

Q. Describe your experience. Does dengue make you feel really awful?

A. The symptoms of dengue fever were so unpleasant that they made a beautiful place like Australia seem unwelcoming. I don't remember being bitten by the dengue mosquito, but I do remember finding a mosquito bite on my neck before I started feeling bad. The dengue mosquito breeds around damp areas, including inside houses, and generally bites people indoors during the day. I was staying at a hotel with friends, and the desk clerk got dengue fever a few days before me, so I believe some dengue mosquitoes were nesting in or near the hotel.

After falling asleep feeling fine, I woke up one night shivering and shaking. I knew I had a fever right away, but it was worse than any other I had ever had. I couldn't sleep the rest of the night because I would feel extremely cold then [really] hot. I began throwing up and experienced diarrhea.

I got up with my friend to see the sunrise thinking I could make it, but I almost fainted just walking to the beach. These were just the initial symptoms, as the next few days would be terrible.

Q. What were your most severe symptoms?

A. The worst symptoms of dengue fever were basically all of them. They included a sudden fever as I previously stated. My temperature rose to 103°F in only a matter of hours. The fever was followed by intense headaches, especially around the eyes. My eyes hurt so bad, I would move my entire head to look around as I couldn't move my eyes due to the extreme pain. I also had muscle and joint pain, especially in my legs. A nickname for the disease is "breakbone" because it feels like your bones are breaking. I ate close to nothing for a few days due to a lack of appetite and terrible taste in my mouth that made even water taste bad. After a few days of those symptoms, a rash began on my legs, and the only good thing about it was that it signaled the end of the virus. During the entire virus, I was also extremely fatigued. I had zero energy, as going to the bathroom was a challenging task. I lost about fifteen pounds due to the virus as well.

Q. How long were you sick?

A. The major symptoms last about eight days, but I felt the aftereffects for approximately one month.

Q. What was the worst thing about dengue fever?

A. I had to fly home with dengue fever feeling like I was going to die. The flight was eighteen hours long, and our plea for a first-class seat failed. I must have gone to the bathroom a record number of times for one flight, and when we landed, my concerned mom was waiting for me at the gate with a wheelchair. I declined the wheelchair because I figured I had just survived the grueling flight that would never end, so I could surely manage a walk to the car.

Q. Anything else you would like to say about your experience with dengue?

A. Don't get dengue fever!

Treatment and Vaccines

Dengue fever has no cure and no medical course of treatment. When a person falls ill with dengue, there is little doctors can do to help, other than to recommend fluids and rest. Basically, the virus just has to run its course, taking as much time as needed for symptoms to come and go. Often, a person does end up in the hospital so doctors can monitor him or her closely, to make sure his or her health is improving, not worsening.

Ultimately, finding a cure for dengue is the goal, so research for a treatment is ongoing. With dengue fever cropping up all over the world, with bigger infections each year, scientists know the importance of finding a vaccine for the disease. A vaccine is a substance that is administered to produce or artificially increase immunity to a particular disease.

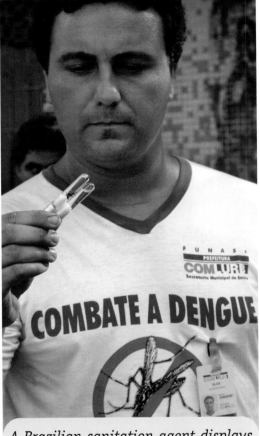

A Brazilian sanitation agent displays a water sample containing mosquito larvae, which may be contaminated.

Finding a vaccine for dengue is proving to be difficult. The fact that dengue has four different serotypes makes vaccination research a bit more tricky. The vaccine must create immunity for all four serotypes. Remember how dengue serotypes are incredibly similar but also very unique? Scientists are having a hard time finding one vaccine that works on all four.

Right now, possible dengue vaccines are being tested in Thailand at Mahidol University with the support of the WHO's regional office for Southeast Asia. The most exciting news is that scientists are making progress. One formulation actually works when given to animals; it is called tetravalent live attenuated vaccine.

It will be years before the vaccine is ready for human testing, but so far the outlook is pretty good. Even with this much achievement, an effective dengue vaccine may not be available to the public for five to ten years.

Emergency Preparation and Response

Mark Bender makes a great suggestion when he says no one should get dengue fever. Think of how tough his experience was and then multiply his experience by thousands of people. Imagine being a doctor and trying to help thousands of dengue patients, knowing there is no cure and no truly effective medicine. Imagine how the government is going to respond. Dengue outbreaks are demanding, complex situations, and many times they do not have easy solutions.

In fact, one of the biggest challenges faced by health officials is how to handle an outbreak of dengue fever. *Dengue and Dengue Hemorrhagic Fever in the Americas:*

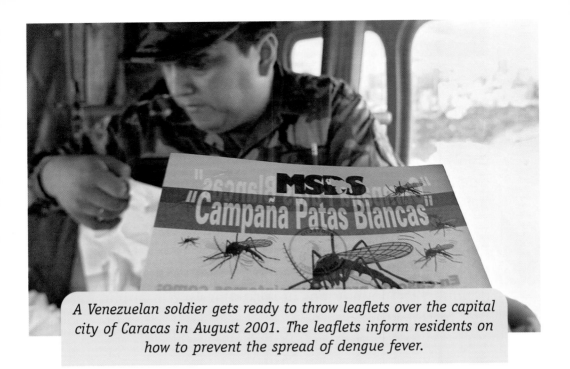

A Venezuelan soldier gets ready to throw leaflets over the capital city of Caracas in August 2001. The leaflets inform residents on how to prevent the spread of dengue fever.

Guidelines for Prevention and Control, a book published by the Pan American Health Organization, suggests the problem begins early on, because "dengue outbreaks are frequently not recognized as such until cases reach into the thousands." This immediately sets health officials far behind in the fight because they are up against thousands of infections, rather than a few hundred. This means more scientists, more doctors, more money, and more planning—all of which are usually lacking in an emergency response to a dengue outbreak. Fortunately, things are changing as countries become more aware of the incredible risks of being unprepared. So, how can a country prepare for a dengue outbreak?

Form an Emergency Committee

According to *Dengue and Dengue Hemorrhagic Fever in the Americas: Guidelines for Prevention and Control*, every country should form an emergency committee that concentrates on dengue fever. This committee, made up of scientists and health and government officials, should meet before an outbreak occurs. Then, if an outbreak does happen, the country is already prepared.

The committee should have a variety of important tasks, but researching the country's dengue control program would be its largest responsibility. Most countries have an existing dengue control program that offers methods of prevention, as well as the proposed response of government and health officials during an outbreak. These emergency committees are also in charge of making sure the dengue control program is effective once an outbreak has occurred—does the country have enough dengue-educated personnel, enough insecticides to spray, and enough mosquito equipment? What is the country's ability to respond to an outbreak?

Many questions should be asked and all of them need to be answered, because if one strategy is not fully prepared or understood, a dengue outbreak may become worse with more people becoming infected.

Along these same lines, the committee should have a country map that shows high-risk areas; those areas should be tested periodically to catch an outbreak early on.

Issuing an Alert

What if an outbreak actually happens? What kind of emergency response can the public expect? Will there be instructions for the public and for medical personnel?

Actually, even before an outbreak is declared, most countries issue an alert. The alert means that an outbreak is imminent. The alert is usually posted on the country's official Web site, run in newspapers, and relayed on television.

Keep in mind, though, that what qualifies as a threatening situation for one country may not be considered dangerous for another. This depends on many factors, such as whether the country has seen dengue fever before or what the climate is like. The following three factors may alert an imminent outbreak:

- Increased number of dengue infections
- An epidemic in a nearby country
- Discovering new dengue cases with a serotype the country has never seen before

Declaring an Emergency

Dengue and Dengue Hemorrhagic Fever in the Americas: Guidelines for Prevention and Control states, "the criteria for determining whether a situation is an emergency varies from country to country and from one year to the next in each country." Similar to when a country decides whether to issue an alert, declaring an emergency also depends on a variety of factors. If a country has never before seen dengue and infection occurs, then that country may choose to declare an emergency rather quickly. If a country has had many epidemics, then that country may not wish to declare an emergency and inform the public right away. But once an emergency is declared, there are several actions that must be followed.

Entering the Emergency Phase

Once an alert has been issued and an emergency declared, a country moves into the emergency phase. The most vital aspect of this phase is communication: Government and health officials must discuss all of their decisions. Next comes gathering, which means gathering supplies, human resources, medical personnel, and any necessary equipment. The emergency committee should give a report that features the map of the country, showing high-target areas or where most people are sick.

Then comes response, which means the emergency plan is being executed. This ranges from increasing medical staff at hospitals to working on killing off the breeding mosquitoes in the high-target areas and surrounding areas. Eradication usually involves insecticides, which are chemicals sprayed into the air to kill the infected mosquitoes. Most importantly, the community must be kept informed of the outbreak, as well as how it can get involved in helping.

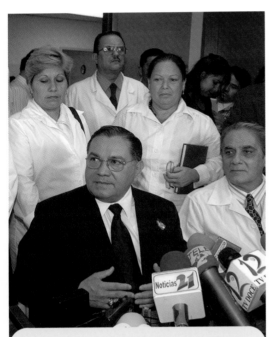

The minister of health of El Salvador, Jose Lopez, holds a press conference on measures to fight dengue fever.

Community Response

During an outbreak or a declared emergency, the community has a very important role. First, the members of the community must remain calm. Overreacting to an outbreak can breed negative consequences, like excessive fear and

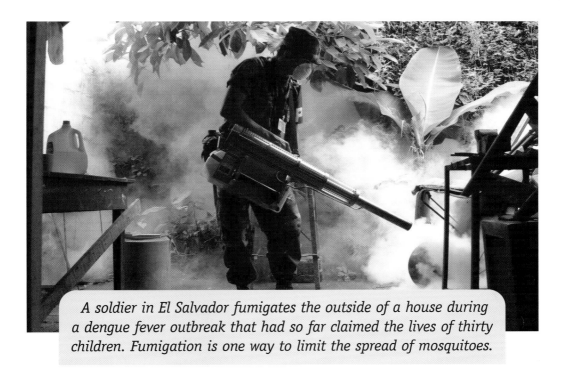

A soldier in El Salvador fumigates the outside of a house during a dengue fever outbreak that had so far claimed the lives of thirty children. Fumigation is one way to limit the spread of mosquitoes.

sometimes even violence. There is no need to overreact. There is a large need for education and learning. Learning what each person can do to help control the outbreak is the best response that can come from the community. Emptying any containers filled with rainwater and getting rid of any trash in or around the home are two great ways to help out government officials and the medical community. Volunteering to educate others and helping others get rid of trash and water-filled containers are also positive steps toward controlling an outbreak.

Although a country should plan well for an outbreak, it should devote even more time, people, and energy toward prevention. Since there is no cure yet for dengue fever, prevention is most certainly the way of the future. Prevention is proactive because it works to decrease the likelihood of an outbreak by controlling the environmental factors that increase dengue fever. Prevention also controls the breeding of mosquito populations. Overall, prevention is the best way to combat dengue fever.

4

PREVENTION AND THE FUTURE

With two-fifths of the world's population at risk and 100 countries already infected with dengue fever, finding and finishing a vaccine is top priority. But while scientists are looking for that vaccine, something must be done to control dengue fever. This is where prevention and control become major influences in the fight against dengue.

Prevention is when a country cuts down on the risk of dengue fever through preventative actions. Control is a by-product of that prevention; through prevention a country can control the risk of dengue outbreaks. Back in the 1960s, when dengue-infested countries around the world made prevention their biggest goal, many were successful and actually eradicated the threatening *Aedes aegypti* mosquito. Why then is dengue back on the rise? What went wrong with prevention?

47

Looking Back to Learn

That's exactly what scientists wanted to know, so they began to study the old prevention programs. Below is what they came up with:

- Not all of the countries joined the eradication efforts, and those that didn't eventually reinfected the newly eradicated ones.

- Dengue programs lost political importance only a few years after they began.

- Often, the response to eradicate dengue was too late to stop reinfestation.

By studying the old eradication programs, scientists learned that eradication is not necessarily the best way to go. Instead, countries should focus on prevention and control. But how does a country actually prevent dengue fever? Isn't that the big question all the scientists want to answer, so they can cut down on the disease?

The fact is, not one country has perfected dengue prevention. Part of this has to do with the fact that every country will need a unique prevention program because every country has a different environment for dengue. For some it could have more to do with climate, while for others a bad waste management system could make for great mosquito breeding. Scientists and health organizations have come up with some very important guidelines for dengue prevention. Getting countries to put them into action may be an altogether different challenge.

New Prevention Actions

In June 1999, the Pan American Health Organization released new information about the best way to control and prevent dengue. In a *Blueprint for Action for the Next Generation: Dengue Prevention and Control*, PAHO cites four actions that can help fight dengue fever.

Action 1

To promote the participation of individuals, families, and communities in dengue prevention and control activities. The goal is to eliminate *Aedes aegypti* breeding sites in and around the home, workplace, and leisure sites.

Action 2

To promote and reinforce changes in human behavior through health communication and health strategies. This includes participation from schools to mass media. The plan is to reach most of the population and affect the society as a whole.

Action 3

To promote and strengthen dengue surveillance at the local level, and to determine *Aedes aegypti* breeding and the amount of infestation. Detecting areas of new infestation and taking necessary actions to prevent further spread of the mosquito are also on the agenda.

Action 4

To strengthen early detection of dengue cases and rapid control measures and to reduce transmission and prevent the occurrence of epidemics.

Mosquito Prevention and Control

Although the PAHO actions may sound a bit official, their main point is very important: People and the government need to take action against dengue and build prevention programs. Then, dengue prevention programs *must* be followed.

According to the American Mosquito Control Association, prevention programs are divided into two areas of responsibility: the individual and the public. These programs are often built on environmental conditions,

According to Rutgers University, mosquitoes have a few favorite places to live. One of these places is in running water. A few mosquito species breed in running water, like streams and creeks. But the young mosquito is easily killed when streams rush after rain.

Transient water is another place mosquitoes enjoy. Transient water is flooded areas, snowpools, and ditches. These are big breeding grounds for *Aedes aegypti*. Transient water lasts for only short periods of time, like a few weeks or a few months. Permanent water, also called semi-permanent water, is another favorite place for mosquitoes. Permanent water is around longer than transient water and often grows plants and water vegetation. Cattails, rushes, and sedges are typical freshwater swamp vegetation. Containers are another favorite place. Container water habitats can be found in natural or manmade settings, such as water held by plants to the water found in tires. Artificial containers are one of the most popular ways for the mosquito to be carried out of its natural environment to a new location.

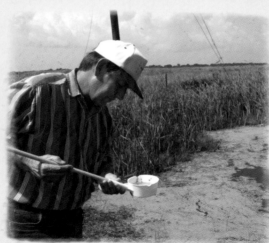

A mosquito control director checks water for mosquito larvae in Louisiana.

money and finances, and social factors. The programs are intended to cut down on dengue infections and improve the quality of life of the people who live in the area.

The Government's Role

While one individual can prevent dengue fever for himself or herself and his or her family, one person cannot prevent dengue fever for everyone. Instead, dengue prevention must be a group effort, something for which a community and city take action.

Government, whether city, state, or country, must also organize mosquito prevention programs. The American Mosquito Control Association states that permanent measures include impounding water and draining swampy mosquito breeding areas. This leaves mosquitoes with nowhere to breed in large numbers. More temporary measures are spraying insecticides with trucks or airplanes. The goal of spraying is to kill adult and larval mosquitoes. Killing larvae is one of the most effective ways to control mosquito populations.

Mechanical Barriers

Keeping windows closed or having tight screens on open windows is one of the most simple and easy ways to keep mosquitoes out. Remember, mosquitoes breed best in hot weather, which also happens to be when windows are left open to let in a breeze. At the beginning of summer, it's a good idea to check all of the windows for screens and to make sure those screens do not have any holes.

Repellents

Repellents are substances that make a mosquito avoid biting people. Many times, people who live in places with high mosquito populations wear repellent when they go outdoors. Perhaps you have worn repellent when you've gone camping?

Overall, repellent prevents mosquito bites because of certain chemicals that fend off the bug. When choosing a repellent, always look for small amounts of the

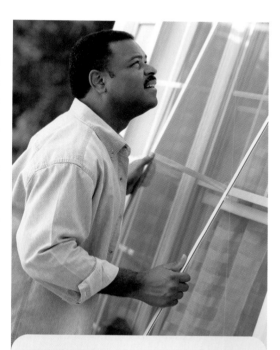

Keeping mosquitoes outdoors by securing windows, doors, and screens is an effective way to prevent dengue fever.

following ingredients: diethyl phthalate, diethyl carbate, N-Diethyl-3-Methylbenzamide (DEET), and ethyl hexanediol. DEET is the most common. If you don't like sprays, mosquito repellent also comes in creams.

Oil of citronella is another type of mosquito repellent. Oil of citronella is often used in outdoor candles. The smoke actually repels the mosquito.

Bug Zappers and Mosquito Traps

The American Mosquito Control Association also suggests mosquito trapping devices and mosquito insect electrocutors (bug zappers) as a way to control mosquitoes around the home. Both are more modern ways of controlling mosquitoes. However, because they are more modern, there is little research on how effective they are. Bug zappers and mosquito traps are more expensive than repellent and citronella candles, but they are supposed to be effective against large amounts of mosquitoes.

Space Sprays

Space sprays are indoor repellents that immediately kill the mosquito. They work best in small areas when windows are closed. For example, a whole house could not be kept mosquito free with space spray. But for problematic areas, space spray is a quick, easy way to kill mosquitoes.

The Future of Dengue Fever

As you know, killing mosquitoes and, on a larger scale, eradication programs, are just not enough to prevent dengue fever all over the world. Remember some of the statistics mentioned in this book? The WHO warns that there are 50 million cases of dengue a year. Almost 2.5 billion people in 100 countries are at risk of getting dengue—that's 40 percent of the world's population. Hopefully, you now understand why scientists have led more studies and why their findings have created even more action. With each study and each new prevention program, doctors, scientists, and government officials learn more about dengue. Look at how the whole concept of the eradication program has changed because of experimentation. Studying what really works to control the spread of dengue has led to more knowledge, so even more effective prevention programs have been designed.

Undoubtedly, dengue fever will continue to make the news. Hopefully, proper prevention programs and an abundance of teamwork will continue to control dengue fever. That will mean one less infection, one less out-break, and one less headline. Scientists all over the world do hope for one headline: "Dengue Vaccine Found." Until that day comes, we must increase our knowledge and take action to control dengue fever.

GLOSSARY

epidemic A disease that affects a large number of individuals within a population, community, or region at the same time.

eradication Destroying the elements needed to house or create a disease, virus, or infection.

dengue fever An incurable, mosquito-borne virus that affects tropical climates; although not fatal, symptoms include a high fever, painful body aches, skin rashes, and bleeding.

dengue hemorrhagic fever (DHF) A more severe form of dengue fever, that can be fatal.

hemorrhagic manifestations Areas on the skin or in the blood vessels that weaken because of illness and begin to leak or bleed; bruising easily is a sign of hemorrhaging.

immunity When a person cannot become infected with a virus because he or she has already carried it.

incubation period Time from the moment of exposure to the development of the symptoms of a disease.

insecticide A chemical sprayed into the air that kills mosquitoes.

outbreak A sudden rise in the incidence of a disease.

pandemic When a disease spreads over a wide geographic area and affects an exceptionally high number of people.

taxonomy A system of classification that compares one disease to another, so doctors, scientists, and medical experts can understand how every disease is similar to and different from one another.

transmission When a virus, disease, or infection is being passed on or spread to someone else.

vaccine A substance that is administered to produce or artificially increase immunity to a particular disease.

virus serotype Scientific term for closely related viruses that share similarities.

FOR MORE INFORMATION

Centers for Disease Control and Prevention (CDC)
1600 Clifton Road
Atlanta, GA 30333
(404) 639-3311
Web site: http://www.cdc.gov

Environmental Protection Agency (EPA)
Ariel Rios Building
1200 Pennsylvania Avenue NW
Washington, DC 20460
(202) 260-2090
Web site: http://www.epa.gov

Health Canada
A.L. 0900C2
Ottawa, ON K1A 0K9
(800) 267-1245
Web site: http://www.hc-sc.gc.ca

National Institutes of Health (NIH)
9000 Rockville Pike
Bethesda, MD 20892
(301) 496-4000
Web site: http://www.nih.gov

Pan American Health Organization (PAHO)
Regional Office of the World Health Organization
525 Twenty-third Street NW
Washington, DC 20037
(202) 974-3000
Web site: http://www.paho.org/default.htm

World Health Organization (WHO)
Avenue Appia 20
1211 Geneva 27
Switzerland
(+ 41 22) 791-21-11
Web site: http://www.who.int/en
e-mail: info@who.int

Web Sites

Due to the changing nature of Internet links, the
Rosen Publishing Group, Inc., has developed an online
list of Web sites related to the subject of this book.
This site is updated regularly. Please use this link to
access the list:

http://www.rosenlinks.com/epid/defe

FOR FURTHER READING

Bailey, Jill. *Mosquito*. Portsmouth, NH: Heinemann Library, 2001.

Coldrey, Jennifer, and George Bernard. *Mosquito*. Englewood Cliffs, NJ: Silver Burdett Press, 1997.

Day, Nancy. *Malaria, West Nile, and Other Mosquito-Borne Diseases*. Englewood Cliffs, NJ: Enslow Publishers, 2001.

Gibbons, Tony. *Mosquitoes*. Milwaukee, Wisconsin: Gareth Stevens, 1997.

Spielman, Andrew, and Michael D'Antonio. *Mosquito: A Natural History of Our Most Persistent and Deadly Foe*. New York: Hyperion Books, 2001.

Spielman, Andrew, and Michael D'Antonio. *Mosquito: The Story of Man's Deadliest Foe*. New York: Hyperion Books, 2002.

INDEX

CREDITS

About the Author

Katherine White is a freelance writer and editor in and around New York City.

Photo Credits

Designer: Evelyn Horovicz; Editor: Eliza Berkowitz